The Infertility Diaries Bonus Book

Inside the crazy, heartbreaking world of infertility told by
a highly emotional infertility survivor who swears she nearly lost her
mind more than once during her years of suffering with infertility.

The Infertility Diaries Bonus Book
Paula Fuoco Davis
PaulaMediaandEntertainment.com, Nashua, NH
Edition Notice 1
Date of Publication: Nov. 10, 2016
Number of Printings: First printing
Year of publication: 2016

opinion only of the author. It is a work of literature and some of the conversations, quoted dialogue, experiences, statements, opinions, emotions expressed may be works of fiction. Some of the incidents and statements may be imaginary in nature. Parts of this book are to be classified as fiction, created by imagination and not based strictly on history or fact.

By reading this book, you agree to comply with the following:

This book's author, publisher, its affiliates or employees are not to be held responsible for any inaccuracies, omissions, editorial errors or any consequences resulting from the information provided.

This book's author, publisher, its affiliates and employees are not to be held responsible for any inaccuracies, omissions, misquotations in the book, and it will be considered a work of fiction, a piece of literature and a story created by imagination, not based strictly on history or fact.

By continuing to read this book, you indicate acceptance of these terms. Those who do not accept these terms should not read, access, use, interact with, view or listen to this book.

The material within this book is not intended to be a definitive set of instructions. Readers who fail to consult with appropriate health authorities assume the risk of any injuries.

The author and publisher of this book are not responsible for errors or omissions or resulting injury from anything written in this book.

The entire content of this book is not intended as a substitute for a medical diagnosis or treatment by qualified medical professionals. Please consult your physician for personalized medical advice.

Always seek the advice of a qualified healthcare provider with any questions regarding a medical condition, diagnosis, or treatment.

Never disregard or delay seeking professional medical advice or treatment because of something you have read or seen in this book.

mental health professional before making any decision regarding treatment of yourself or others.

If you are currently in treatment or in therapy, please consult your therapist, psychiatrist or mental health professional before you use any of the information contained in this book.

If you feel suicidal or depressed, contact a Crisis Hotline or seek help at a hospital, Emergency Room, treatment center, or with a physician, qualified mental health care provider, or through a law enforcement agency or social services.

This book and its contents (including any information available from the book located on websites or excerpted) is for informational and entertainment purposes only and is not intended to replace or substitute for any professional, medical, legal, mental health or any other advice.

In addition, the author and publisher make no representations or warranties and expressly disclaims any and all liability concerning any treatment or action by any person following the information offered or provided within or through this book. If you have specific concerns or find yourself in a situation in which you require professional or medical advice, you should consult with an appropriately trained and qualified specialist.

Please consult your physician, mental health professional or therapist before you utilize the materials that can be purchased from this book.

If you do not agree to be bound by all of these terms, do not read this book.

We make no representation or warranties with respect to the accuracy or completeness of the contents of the book and we specifically disclaim any implied warranties of merchantability for any particular purpose.

All material in this book is provided for your information only and may not be construed as medical advice or instruction. No action or inaction should be taken based on the contents of this information. Instead, readers should consult appropriate health professionals on any matter relating to their health and well-being.

The information in this book does not and is not intended to replace professional medical or nutritional advice.

The information contained in this book should not be considered complete and does not cover all diseases, ailments, physical conditions or their treatment. It should not be used in place of a call or visit to a medical,health or other competent professional, who should be consulted beforeadopting any of the suggestions in this book or drawing inferences from it.

The information about drugs, herbs, vitamins, foods, drinks, and any other food sources contained in this book is general in nature.

They do not cover all possible uses, actions, precautions, side effects, or interactions of the medicines mentioned, nor is the information intended as medical advice for individual problems or for making an evaluation as to the risks and benefits of taking a particular drug, vitamin, herb, supplement, or food.

This book and the operator(s) of this site specifically disclaim all responsibility for any liability, loss or risk, personal or otherwise, which is incurred as a consequence, directly or indirectly, of the use and application of any of the material on this site.

If you do anything recommended in this book without the supervision of a licensed medical doctor, you do so at your own risk because the information, remedies or exercise in this book may not be U.S. Food and Drug Administration (FDA) approved.

The medical information in this book is provided "as is" without any representations or warranties, express or implied.

You must not rely on the information in this book as an alternative to medical advice from your doctor or other professional health care provider.

If you think you may be suffering from any medical condition or before starting any new treatment you should seek immediate medical attention. Proper medical attention should always be sought for specific ailments.

Never disregard professional medical advice, delay in seeking medical treatment or discontinue medical treatment due to information obtained in this book

Any information provided in this book is not intended to diagnose, treat or cure infertility or any other illness, disease or medical condition.

Books may be purchased by contacting the publisher and author at books@paulamediaandentertainment.com.

Books may be purchased in quantity and/or special sales by contacting the publisher, PaulaMediaandEntertainment.com or by email at books@paulamediaandentertainment.com.

Library of Congress Catalog Number:
ISBN:
   1. Infertility 2. Fertility 3. Health

   First Edition

This book is dedicated to my mother, Sarah Fuoco for being the best mother in the world.

My father, Joseph Fuoco, for being one of the kindest men I ever met.

My beautiful children, Amber and Sammy, who God sent as an answer to all my prayers.

Jehovah God, who gives the privilege of prayer and who is always there.

My best friend, Leah Page Mortimer, who walked with me and helped me every step of the way.

My husband, Christopher Davis, for being there and walking this hard road with me. You were brave and kind, a true hero, and without you, I would not have my kids.

Table of Contents

The Doctor Called My Eggs "Bottom of the Barrel"

My doctor looked at me point blank and said without a trace of mercy that my eggs were "bottom of the barrel."

Bottom of the barrel... Her words rang in my head like a cruel pronouncement.

I was 37 years old and desperately wanted a second child. My doctor didn't believe I could have one.

I had been through this before. To have my daughter, I endured 10 IUIs, several operations and too many nights of crying to count.

So I left her office: desperate, heartbroken, and wildly, frantically panicked. The words 'your eggs are bottom of the barrel' kept repeating in my head. Despite everything I've gone through, I always had hope. My insides were screaming: 'I can't live with this.' I was so shaken, I could barely drive home. Her words nearly broke my will and spirit to try again.

For some reason, on the way home, I stopped at a natural foods market. Walking around the supermarket, amidst all the healthy foods and supplements, I began to question what the doctor told me. Was the poor quality of my eggs something that could be improved? Was I unhealthy on some undetectable level that was impacting my fertility? I went home and called my ever-wise mother. She gave me great advice: dump that doctor and try again.

I did exactly what Mom said. I decided I would do everything I could to restore and heal my fertility, and not be hindered by my age, regardless of what the doctor said.

Over time, I learned that there was hope for me and others like me—and just because a doctor says you can never get pregnant does not mean your body, if given the right elements, cannot heal from infertility.

My devastation and despair turned to determination, and

everything I learned, I put in this book. As a newspaper reporter for more than 25 years, I utilized my skills as a journalist to get to the root of fertility problems, the physical and the emotional.

I am now also a fertility success certified life coach and I wrote about how I healed my body in my book "Dancing Your Way to Fertility" that is also available on Amazon.com. That book includes my story, along with The Ultimate Fertility Success Program which I believe is one of the most comprehensive body-mind makeover plans available to fertility patients today.

The Ultimate Fertility Success Program includes 12 cleanses that will detoxify your body and expand your fertility potential.
It will also show you how to improve the quality of your eggs—something previously not thought possible—and balance your hormones.

In this book, The Infertility Diaries, I share my personal journey of battling infertility, a rotten opponent that needed to be knocked upside its head and kicked to the curb.

It wasn't easy and there were moments, as you will read, that nearly broke me.

That doctor who claimed my eggs were 'bottom of the barrel' was wrong. Less than a year later, I gave birth to my beautiful son.

Someday, I would like to send her a picture of my boy and write in blazing letters across the picture: "Is this what bottom of the barrel looks like?"

This is a condensed version of The Infertility Diaries, which can be purchased at Amazon.com.

The Start of My Journey

Today is my first day of writing a journal on my road to victory over infertility. I am writing this for women like me who have been told that their eggs are too old, that our bodies are too old, weak, or damaged, that there is little hope. I am writing this book for women who feel that having a child is some type of impossible dream, that they are the victim of some pathologically cruel biological problem.

I am writing this book for women who, like me, dream of starting a family, but find the road long, cruel, uphill, and not always forgiving of slight mistakes and accumulated years.

I am 36 years old. Last week, a doctor that seemed very kind when I first met her told me that my eggs were the 'bottom of the barrel.' I have been seething with pain and engulfed in sadness ever since.

'Bottom of the barrel' the very image leaves me feeling hopeless. I cannot yell at her. I cannot criticize her. For if I do, the clinic may label me 'psychologically unfit' to undergo further infertility treatments. So I stay quiet. I watch my words. I must adhere to and accept as normal their warped and perverse idea that pulling hope away is truly in the best interest of the patient, when with all my heart I know that it is only hope and faith that will ultimately give me the baby I so desperately want. What kind of monsters are they? I so want to walk into that clinic, tell that monster doctor disguised as a kind, caring medical professional off, and never step foot in there again. But then what? I have no choice but to bite my tongue, and wait until it is my turn to walk in there with a beautiful baby and say, "hello, do you want to see what bottom of the barrel looks like?' That is when my victory will be complete.

 For now, I wait and suffer and try to erase their hopeless images from my head.

In this book, I will recount my experience with infertility.

I will tell you now that this book will end with my successfully creating the family I dream of.
I say this with confidence, for I believe God created us with a body that

can heal and thrive and grow past illness, and that doctors do not understand the miracle of faith and the miracle of hope.

And for that doctor who tried to destroy my hope, I dedicate this book to you and anyone else who believes in stomping on a women's hope.

I don't always believe in being realistic—in putting my faith in only what I can see. Sometimes holding on to a dream takes being strong enough to push aside the skeptics, the cynics, the naysayers and delving into the world of hope--a world that takes a lot of strength to hold on to when everything around you is crumbling.

I begin this day by swimming. I am trying to get as healthy as possible. In the world of infertility, at 36, I am labeled old, but I don't feel old. Well, yes, maybe I do feel old. Withered inside at times. I just went through a harrowing IVF that ended with my becoming pregnant, only to lose the baby within two weeks of conception.

Cruel. That is how I feel right now about the past two weeks: cruel. They dubbed this pregnancy a chemical pregnancy, relegating it to something that almost didn't happen, didn't really happen, never existed. Thus was taken my right to feel sad or mourn, as it wasn't a pregnancy and it wasn't a miscarriage, but it was in a way, or is it? Nothing...dismiss it...mourning stamped invalid.

Most of all, I dedicate this book to God, who is the strength of my life. Without the privilege of prayer, I could not endure the hell of infertility. When the load was too heavy, it was only through prayer to God that I kept one foot in front of the other and kept trying.

So together, I begin this journey with you, a fellow infertility victim and survivor. I pray that we all see victory, in whatever form we wish it to come. For those of you wanting a child, I pray for your victory.

For those of you who have come to the point that adoption is a joyful option, I pray for you. I pray that we all can have the families we want and deserve, for family is a blessing and a gift, and all women deserve to receive this treasure of security, companionship, love and purpose.

Adjusting To A New Way of Life

In many ways, starting infertility treatments is like starting a new life—one I wasn't exactly ready for. I tip toed into this process, rather than diving headfirst into it. When I first began, I didn't think a lot about what was happening—all I knew is I wanted a baby and I felt safe that I was in the hands of a reputable fertility clinic. I didn't analyze much or have a well thought-out strategy.

I suppose, looking back, my tip toe approach worked for me, but it was not one I had the luxury of staying with for very long.

I was not prepared for how demanding treatments can be...blood tests at 6 a.m., ultrasounds, more blood tests, shots every night. I was often late for my appointments. I had a hard time juggling my work schedule and the demands of the clinic. I had not yet altered my life enough to include fertility. It felt like an interruption I wasn't yet ready to surrender to.

I felt like the clinic was constantly calling me wanting something...another blood test, one more ultra-sound—didn't they realize that if went to the 6:30 a.m. ultrasound, I would be exhausted by the time I got out of work at 9 o'clock?

Surrender...that is the word that describes the process in many ways. Battling infertility takes battling, but it also takes surrender. For someone like me, I had to progress to the point where the requirements of the clinic had to take priority over my own exhaustion, work schedule, social life, or personal desires.

At a certain point, the only personal desire I had to pay attention to was my desire for a baby.

For the first six months, I was consistently late for most of my appointments. I sometimes didn't show up due to my work schedule or car problems. I did this so many times, I finally got called on the carpet by Dr. P.

"Are you ready for this?" he asked. He told me that if I continued to miss appointments or show up late, the clinic could not continue treating me.

Talk about a wake-up call.

Suddenly, I realized that I had to take this whole process very seriously and live up to whatever it was the clinic asked of me, even when it was hard. I could blow my opportunity to have what I most wanted due to my own irresponsible behavior.

I explained to Dr. P some of the problems caused by my work schedule, and a few car problems that caused me to miss appointments.

He understood, but made it clear that this type of behavior couldn't continue and was not acceptable.

If I wanted their help, I had to be responsible. If I wanted these treatments to work, I had to commit to doing whatever they asked. Whenever they wanted me there, I had to be there.

Looking back, I consider this the first step in my training for motherhood: being responsible isn't an option.

I walked out of that appointment somber and scared.

I wanted a baby, and I would have to put aside whatever was preventing me from getting to my appointments on time.

This was one of the many turning points in my treatment.

Dr. P was forcing me to make a choice: continue life as you know it, without 6 a.m. blood tests, or go through this painful, inconvenient, life-interrupting process in order to get what you want most.

I left knowing I had to change, and this was one of the many times my infertility treatments would push me in ways that I needed to be pushed in order to become the mother I wanted to be.

Hard Time of Year

It is the week of Christmas and reminders that I have no children in my life are everywhere I turn.

I have no one to buy toys for, no one to bundle up and take sledding, no one to make hot chocolate for. Everywhere I look, there are commercials with beautiful little girls in pink and white dresses marveling at some wonderful new doll their mother has bought them.

Seeing it dangled before me constantly, I feel far removed from this normal and beautiful part of life.

I go in the Disney store at the mall and I run out almost immediately. When do I get a child to buy toys for? A child to tell whimsical fairy tales to? When does the magic I am seeing and hearing about all the time get to be mine to enjoy?

This feeling culminated when we visited my parents a few days ago for dinner.

I went there feeling depressed. It is December, and I am not pregnant yet. I am surrounded and constantly assaulted by visions of big families with lots of children gathering together. I see these images and ask: will I ever have this or will I always be so alone in this world?

When we got to my parent's house, I was feeling sorry for myself. I couldn't help feeling that this dinner shouldn't be so small.

The feeling was so overwhelming that I made a decision that day: this will be the last December I ever experience without a child in my life. If I don't get pregnant soon, I am going to adopt.

I was feeling pretty down, so I escaped to the upstairs bedroom. My husband followed me and asked what was wrong. I started to cry. He held me, and I told him it hurts so much to not have a baby yet... to month after month not be pregnant.

Just then, my father knocks on the door and wants to know what is wrong. I tell him about how hard it is for me to have yet another December come and go without a child in my life. He looks at me, obviously a bit confused, and says, "Can't we just have a nice day? We don't want the day ruined."

That was it for me. I was feeling very depressed to begin with, but this was too much. I storm downstairs, shouting a few choice words about his insensitivity, and lock myself in the downstairs bathroom.

 I was not coming out until dinner was over and it was time to go home!

At that moment, I was already struggling to fight off my extreme disappointment and I had no stomach for my father's inability to understand the validity of my pain. I felt safer in the bathroom than being with someone who didn't fully get how beaten down a woman can feel when she is ready to welcome new members into her family, and those new members are not arriving as expected.

My mother and husband tried to get me to come out and enjoy dinner, but I just couldn't. I felt ashamed…a total loser…angry..So, so angry. I just wanted to stay hidden.

Maybe this wasn't the most mature response or the most considerate action to take, since my mother worked hard to prepare a lovely meal, but lately my emotions have been building towards a boiling point and once heated, I am unable turn them back.

I have little tolerance for all the people who take my feelings about being childless so lightly.

It seems everywhere I go, no one understands how painful infertility is-- a raw, blistering, heated pain that never lets up.

I need at least my family to understand how bad this feels.

Today I desperately needed them to understand just how hard it is for another family dinner to arrive and still it is just my tiny little family with no children.

Why couldn't my Dad see how hurt I am? How alone I feel? How horrible it is to experience life without a baby to love, when it seems every other family is overflowing with new babies, new children, a never ending supply of new life?

Where are the children who are suppose to be running around our family dinner table? When does new life get to come into our family?

On TV, I am barraged with images of big loving families with lots of adorable little children sitting at long beautifully set tables. I need that in my life.

I live in a dead zone with everything so stagnant and unchanging.

I need new babies at our family dinner table. I don't want another family dinner with the same cast of characters.

Give me new life, give me babies.

I want my Dad and everyone else to know that I feel like the loneliest freak in the world because I am without children. I feel like life is passing by me. Somehow, along the way, I got on the wrong track and something I was suppose to have has been stolen away.

I hurt so much. It was impossible for me to come out of the bathroom and pretend everything is fine. Nothing is fine.

It felt a lot less painful to lock myself in the bathroom than experience another family dinner with no children.

Chris eats quickly, thanks my mother, and we leave.

A Few Days Later

Now that a few days have passed, I understand a bit more clearly where my father was coming from when he said 'can't we just have a nice day.' He was excited to have us over for a visit and he wanted enjoy a good time. No dramatics. Just a quiet enjoyable dinner with his family.

He probably doesn't understand what the big deal is about having kids, especially since he only had me and what I have been to him is mostly trouble and upset. It must be very difficult for a logical man like my father to have a daughter like me--dramatic, sensitive, super emotional, always ready to launch into an emotional tirade about this or that.

Normally, my father is an incredibly loving man, but perhaps this time, he just didn't feel like dealing with my issues (trust me, over the years I have had a lot of them.) Maybe for once he wanted things to be easy, pleasant, simple. I can't say I blame him. Easy, pleasant and simple are words that do not in any way describe me.

I know he meant no harm. Still..I'll get over it. He's my Dad. He calls and apologies. A very nice apology. I accept and we make up.

But I meant it when I said this will be the last December I ever experience without a child in my life.

A Visit to the Nutritionist

I decide to get an appointment with an iridologist/nutritionist in Maine. I want to compliment my infertility treatments with holistic medicine so I can get to the root of my problem.

The nutritionist/iridologist is named Sarah M. and she comes highly recommended. She spends almost three hours with me. She starts by analyzing my body through iridology, which is taking an x-ray of my eye and looking at what it tells about my body. She asks me lots of questions. I tell her that I have no energy.

Sometimes, by 1 o'clock in the afternoon, even if I've done nothing all morning, I am exhausted and just want to watch TV in bed.

She recommends a large number of vitamins and herbs. Since I can only afford to buy about five bottles, I ask her what are the top five supplements I need. She said not to worry: my father had called ahead and offered to pay for everything. That's my Dad for you—always so generous and obviously very sorry that he hurt my feelings a few weeks ago. I was so surprised and relieved—now I could get all the vitamins and herbs I needed! It seems my liver, blood and colon all need cleansing. I went home with about 15 bottles. I didn't even want to look at the bill since I felt so guilty that my Dad was paying. I know he spent a lot.

Shivering At Night

It is now the third day on Sarah's program and every night, I shiver in bed for hours before falling asleep. I know all the herbs and vitamins are cleaning me out in some way, removing toxins from my body, but it still feels horrible.

Very, Very Sad

It is June. One year and three months since I began infertility treatments. Such a long time and still no baby. I am sad. No, I am beyond sad--I am enraged, frustrated, full of yearning.

I am tired of yearning.

I long to hold hands with a baby...a baby that is mine.

I look at mothers in supermarkets, mothers who look angry, tired and annoyed at their rambunctious little brats and I think: God, why can't that be me? Why can't I be pushing around a cart full of loud, overtired, rambunctious children?

These mothers look so overworked, and yet they have no idea that I would do anything to have what they have.

These women look deceivingly ordinary in so many ways, and I think:

why can't I have their ordinary life--the one that includes a grocery cart full of babies?

There is a woman I see occasionally who has four young children. She is beautiful and her children are lovely too.

When I saw her holding hands with one of her young sons the other day, I was struck with that image--the image of a woman holding hands with her son.

Hands to hold. I want little hands to hold.

When I see the little hands of a baby, I think: what in the world must it feel like to hold the little hands of a baby that you gave birth to? What I would give to hold such little hands, to know those hands were mine to hold, to know that those were the hands of my daughter or my son?

I am going to write Dr. P a letter to ask that he do a lapascropy to see if I have a problem with endometriosis. I hope he listens and does what I want. I have to word the letter in a way that will get him to do as I ask.

I need little hands to hold. Hands that are all mine. To all the women I see shopping in supermarkets, who see themselves as ordinary mothers, I say--you have everything I want and there is nothing ordinary about your role as the mother to those little humans who are driving you crazy.

Please God, give me a little human to tire me out. Please let me be an ordinary mother in a supermarket one day.

I can't imagine anything in this world more special or more fun than pushing around my babies at the supermarket. My happy-ever-after is so plain and ordinary, boring even, and yet it feels so hopelessly impossible and faraway.

Meeting with Dr. P

I met with Dr. P today and found out a few disturbing things.

One is that yes, he knew I should be moving on to a stronger medicine, but because I tend to get scared and stressed during the procedures, he didn't think I could handle moving on to shots. I want to scream at him!

Instead, I force myself to stay calm and I explain to him that the more time that passes, the less nervous I am during procedures.

He seems skeptical, but I continue talking calmly, stating that while I may seem nervous, that is just my style of coping—and that the moment I leave the clinic, I feel completely calm and back to normal (which is true. I expulse everything and then I'm over it. It could be called being Italian, but I don't say that because it may sound weird.) He agrees to do the lapascropy and will schedule it soon. After that is done, depending on the outcome of the surgery, we will move on to shots. I am now waiting for a surgery date.

The Donut Incentive

They have ordered some new tests. This morning I was scheduled for a test I am dreading. I am so afraid of this particular test.

I don't think I have it in me to do this test. The whole drive down to the clinic, anxiety rattled around my body. How in the world am I going to make myself go through this test?

Then I got an idea: on the way to the clinic, I went to a drive-through Dunkin Donuts and ordered two of my favorite chocolate frosted donuts.

I get to the clinic, sit in the waiting room holding my donut bag, and soon am called in for the test. The nurse leaves the room while I change. When she comes back in, I am lying on the table, dressed in a johnny, with the donut bag sitting on my stomach.

"What are the donuts for?" she asks, straining to act like no-big-deal-so-what-if-a-bag-of-donuts-is-sitting-on-a-patient, but since she's not a professional actress, her irritation comes shining through.

"They are my reward for going through this test," I said.

My logic here is this: if I can lay here, endure whatever I have to endure, all the while seeing and smelling these two donuts that I am going to eat the moment the test is done, the test won't feel so bad or be so hard to take.

Nothing is a better reward for me than chocolate donuts.

The doctor comes in, and very politely asks if I want to eat the donuts sitting on my stomach before they do the test.

Again, he is trying to be nice, but obviously is a bit confused by the presence of the donut bag on my stomach. The great efforts everyone went through to show respect to me, even though I obviously looked eccentric, was both hilarious and touching.
What a nice group of people at this clinic.

"No," I giggled. "I'll eat them later," and it felt good to laugh and see the humor in this whole situation.

They did the test, and all the time I kept focusing on was: if I can get through this test, I can eat my donuts. I tried to think of nothing else, not the pain, not the nurses, not anything but the reward coming: the donuts.

How I love chocolate donuts.

The test ended. Everyone left the room. Before I even changed out of the johnny, I devoured the donuts in about ten seconds.

Ah, the power of chocolate donuts.

Even the most unpleasant test was bearable because I had two grand and delicious donuts to look forward to. Maybe I'll try this again.

Teaching Experience

I have one more IUI before my surgery in July. How great it would be if I got pregnant this time and never had to go through the surgery at all. Today I taught a magazine writing class at the community college I attended in the early 1980s. Since I am a reporter, teaching writing is something I do occasionally.

Typically, I love teaching. I teach one-day classes on Saturdays. Sometimes I teach journalism, sometimes writing your family history, sometimes magazine writing. Usually, teaching these classes leaves me with a buzz, a thrill, a high almost.

When I teach, I am seventeen and in love, I am six and allowed to go on the merry-go-round one more time, I am 11 years old and sitting in my treehouse, I am 14 and someone (anyone) thinks I am pretty.

When I teach, the insecure, negative, self-hating part of me disappears and I emerge strong, confident, and full of possibilities. The girl in college who wore a white cotton dress and truly believed that anything and everything was possible returns briefly for an encore.

When I teach, I realize that my true calling was not working as a newspaper reporter, but being in a classroom with students.

But today, my teaching experience was completely different than usual and left me feeling pretty hysterical. Here's why.

The class started out as usual.

First, I introduce myself, and then I call each student up to my desk to talk one-on-one about why they took the class and what they hope to learn from the class.

The students come to my desk one at a time and share their goals for the class.

Now it is the turn of the woman sitting in the front row who looks to be in her mid-30s. Immediately, I like her. She seems spunky.

Then she opened her mouth, "I'm here to write about my seven year hell with infertility."

Wham--I am in for quite a ride.

For the next seven hours, eight counting lunch, all I hear about is her horrible experience with infertility and how it DIDN'T work out.

Her voice and desire to share her story was louder and more fervent than any other person in class. She had enough anger and fury to dominate the entire class discussion.

"The clinic tricked me."

"I tried everything and it didn't work."

"I'm trying Reiki now, hoping maybe that will work."

"All my husband and I ever wanted was children."

Even during lunch, when I hoped for a break from hearing about her pain, which scarily mirrored my own, she sat with me outside on the picnic bench and continued her story.

I felt for this woman. At another time, the teacher part of me might have been glad she took my class in order to share her pain.

But the infertility patient part of me wanted to tell her to shut up.

I struggled all day to remain professional, calm and not interject with my own experiences with infertility....but inside I was screaming was IS THIS GOING TO BE IN SEVEN YEARS? Am I going to turn into her eventually? Will I try and try like she did and never get a baby? Was her lot my lot? No, no, no, I kept saying to myself. I won't make the same mistakes she made. I was going to a highly reputable clinic. I was already working on improving my overall health.

But still....I felt panicked and scared. Hearing her story just confirmed all my worst fears: that I could do infertility treatments year after year after year with no result.

All she ever wanted was a baby. All I ever wanted was a baby. Were we two peas in the same hopeless pod?

I hid my feelings all day, knowing it would open a can of worms if I told her I too was in the midst of fertility treatments.

But now back at home, I am burning with pain. Will this be me in seven years?

She reminded me yet again of the terrible statistic that not everyone who goes to a fertility clinic ends up with a baby.
I can't stand to hear these statistics. They make me crazy.

I can't go seven more years without a child in my life. I won't be her, because if I don't get pregnant in one year, I will adopt.

I will always and forever keep trying for my own biological baby, but I will adopt before I let seven years pass without a child in my life. Hell, if I end up with both an adopted baby and a biological baby, what an incredible blessing that would be.

Everywhere I turn right now, I feel I am confronted with one hopeless infertility story after another.

Throughout the class, her pain was raw and rageful in a way I clearly understood, but surely didn't want to see, hear or understand. Why did she have to take my class? Was I suppose to hear something she said?

Was I suppose to know that sometimes this doesn't work out?

God help this woman, God help me. Let us both get the babies we so desperately want.

A Door Opens...

Lately, I'm realizing that to get pregnant, I need to get as healthy as I can. When I first started infertility treatments, I thought that infertility medicine alone would do the trick. Then I thought doing an IUI would guarantee a baby.

Now, I am beginning to see that more is needed to make this all work.

Today at work, I started feeling so nervous and desperate that I prayed all day for answers. Every spare minute I could, I asked God to help me give my body whatever it needs to get pregnant. I prayed repeatedly that God would help me get as healthy as I can be.

I feel so afraid that even with everything I am doing, it won't work out.

After work, I went to pick up Chris at the salon where he works as a massage therapist on Saturday.

I've driven that road dozens of times before, so it was odd that today, I noticed a sign I never noticed before: 'Chinese Herbalist'.

Something in me felt compelled to stop. I had recently read that Chinese herbs are sometimes used to help prepare the body for pregnancy. Maybe it wasn't an accident that my eyes landed straight on that sign, especially since I prayed so hard this morning.

I had to stop and see what this herbalist had to say about my condition, especially since I still had a few hours before my husband got off work.

Dr. Myung Kim would turn out to be an answer to my prayer. He turned out to also be an acupuncturist, and while he did not want to sell me any herbs, he recommended acupuncture. I tried acupuncture before and believe in it strongly.

He read my pulse, and told me that I had a weak gallbladder channel. I made my first appointment. He has even written a book on acupuncture.

It turns out that he has a second one about 15 minutes from my home, which I don't think is an accident considering how much I prayed this morning.

Although I have driven down this road about 100 times in the past year, I noticed his storefront today for the first time. Acupuncture needs to be part of my treatment, I am sure of it.

A Moment In Song

Something wildly odd and beautiful happened this afternoon in the parking lot at the supermarket. I was there to meet a friend for coffee, and arrived a little early. Stuck with about an hour to kill, I decided to just listen to the radio.

I started praying about having a baby, as I usually do whenever I have a spare moment.

While I was doing that, Will Smith's "Just The Two of Us" came on the radio. The song is a father singing to his son. The Dad gives his son advice about not swearing, remembering to say your prayers, and holding the door open for girls. I love this song, as you can feel the power of this father's love for his child.
As I listened to the song, a wave of joy came over me--like someday I would actually be able to sing this song to my child.

I imagined that on my child's wedding day, I would play this for him or her, and recount this moment in the parking lot where I was begging for his/her birth.

It wouldn't matter if my child was a boy or a girl--this song would still apply. "Just the Two of Us"--me and my child. I got so deeply into this vision, of me dancing and singing this song to my child at their wedding, that it began to feel completely real. Of course I will have a baby someday! No doubt..it will come to pass...

The song moved me to another time and place, and it felt so completely real, that it was as if it had already happened.

By the end of the song, I was on a wild high, visions of my child dancing in my head: their wedding, their birth, this song being our song. For a few minutes, I landed in such a place of hope.

A good place...

For those few minutes, all the desperation I usually feel was swept away by a tidal wave of faith and hope.

Do I dare think this song was maybe a kind of answer to my prayer?

For a few minutes even after the song ended, a feeling of certainty that I would have a child was mine, all mine.

My prayer, coupled with that song, brought me to a place of joy I haven't felt in a long time.

My child was real--our relationship was real--the future with my child in it all became real.

Could this be a signal? I can't imagine the fullness I will someday feel if there was a little person on this earth I could actually sing and dedicate this song to.

Needing Validation

Everywhere I go, everything I do, in every conversation I have, I am looking for validation that yes, I am someday going to have a baby. I search conversations for clues, for hope, for someone to say "yes you Paula are going to have a baby."

People don't realize how their subtle words and expressions tell me volumes about what they really think about my quest to have a baby. A slight hesitation, a barely detected pause, the way they might casually say having kids is really no big deal, can send me plunging into a wordless, motionless depression.

I am sensitive to the little nuisances in conversation that indicate the person doesn't really think a baby will ever come to me. I see it in that sort of shrugging expression people give when we get on the subject.

I need people to believe in me. I need friends to come right out and say: 'Yes You Can and Will Have a Baby!"

I want people around me to have no qualms about saying the most optimistic thing they can imagine saying to me.

I am hurt by all the people who see me as yet another statistic who won't get pregnant. The other day I was at the doctor's office getting a blood test when I came across an article on infertility and all the article did was rant on and on about the low success rate of infertility patients.

Why did they have this article available to all of us right their in the waiting room, while we are trying so hard despite the odds to get pregnant? Was it there to taunt and torment us?

I don't want to hear those statistics! I am tired of people imagining me a failure before I am ready to see myself that way.

One day at work, out of the blue, my dear friend Judy looked over at me and said, "I picture you with a curly-haired little girl." Imagine...out of the clear blue, she gifted me with a miraculous picture of hope! Judy sees me with a curly-haired daughter!

Does she know how much hope her words gave me that day? Does she know that her words released me from my sadness that day? Does anyone know how good it feels to know that someone else on this earth actually believes in my ability to give birth?

Why aren't more people like Judy? Why do so many people find it easier to believe I will never have a baby?

Lately, some people look at me like a lost cause. I am so tired of people who feel the need to share with me story after story of this person or that person who never could have children. Do people want to see me fail? Do they feel more secure in sharing bad news with me?
Have they seen so much failure and disappointment in their own lives

and in other people's lives, that they no longer believe a person can want something very badly and actually get it?

I don't know why their opinion means so much to me. I shouldn't need their validation so much. I know I shouldn't care what other people think, but I do.

I care because deep down, I agree with them: I don't believe in myself either.

A part of me feels this journey is going to be like lots of the other journeys in my life: me digging and digging for something, trying and trying, only to end up nowhere, and all my effort for nothing.

There is a part of me that has long believed my lot in life was to work and work for things, and end up with nothing. A part of me feels very comfortable on this path right now--doing lots of things without great hope or belief of ever reaping any reward for my efforts.

Many times in my life, almost reaching my goal has felt almost enough for me.

But this time, it has to be different. 'Almost' having a baby, 'almost' being pregnant doesn't count. When I was younger, sometimes I was content with 'almost'.

I even found comfort in all the 'almost' in my life--I almost finished my book for young people when I was in my 20s, I almost had my children's book published, I 'almost' married a man I had adored for years.

Almost felt comfortable--like that was all I deserved. This time, 'almost' can't be good enough--because the reality is, when I am 80 years old, there will be no 'almost baby' sitting beside me. I can't 'almost' be a mother and 'almost' have a baby. This time, I have to go all the way.

God, I want a child so badly. I want to love a little person so much. Will I work and work for this and never see any results for all my efforts?

I need people to believe in me, because I don't believe in myself. I need people to help me silence all the voices in my head telling me this won't work out.

Sometimes, I don't think I am normal enough to have a baby, which is suppose to be the most normal thing in the world for a woman to do.

Getting pregnant and having a baby seem the natural right for other women--women who are better, stronger, more deserving than me.

I seem doomed not to have the ordinary things other women have. I'm not quite sure why, but I've long felt this. Things other women get easily and take for granted seem nearly impossible for me.

I wish I could say to everyone around me: please, tell me I am going to have a baby. Don't be afraid to be crazily-over-the-top-optimistic about my chances.

Don't feed me any more reality stories about friends who tried for years to get pregnant and failed. Don't--please, please don't--tell me that God might have other plans for me. I don't want other plans. I can't see why God wouldn't want me to have a baby. Please don't speak for God and please don't assume that He is always ready to deny me what I want. Believe in me. Hope with me. Kick the odds and the statistics out and see me giving birth. And please, don't tell me life can still be enjoyed without children.

For once, I wish people would err on the side of optimism. I want people to believe in me. Please everybody, tell me lies even. Even if you don't believe in my ability to have a child, lie to me and pretend you do. Tell me I am definitely going to get pregnant.

Hope Comes

It has been three days since I arrived at my parent's house. I still feel very weak. I pray constantly. Having a baby feels like such a faraway dream, just another thing I'm shooting for that I probably won't get.

Prayer gives me hope, despite these negative feelings. If God could open the Red Sea, if He could save Daniel from the lion's den, if He could break down the walls of Jericho, I do believe He can help me. From this, I draw strength.

Today Leah and I went out to do a few errands. We ended up at Wal-Mart, where she needed to pick up some film for her upcoming cross-country trip.

While we were in the photo department, I spot a cute little photo album for babies that said on the cover, "Memories of First Summer." Leah caught me looking at it.

"Buy it," she said.

"Why?" I asked.

"Because next summer you will be using it," she said. Leah is always so encouraging, so positive. She is helping me believe that someday I will definitely have a baby.

"Paula, you need to buy this," she said again.

So, diving into her optimism, I bought it.

I will always be grateful to Leah for this moment, when she took my hand and helped me see a brighter moment ahead, when with my own eyes, it was hard to hope.

Leah and I have been here before. About seven years ago, I was extremely depressed over a bad break-up, an engagement gone wrong. One afternoon, we were sitting on the couch talking, surrounded by a bunch of lace and wedding veil that a friend of hers gave her after closing a wedding business. Suddenly, Leah walked over and placed the veil on me and insisted that I stand up and look in the mirror. "No," I kept refusing, wanting that veil off, because seeing myself ever getting married seemed impossible at that point. She persisted. Finally, I stood up and looked in the mirror, "I am going to see a happy ending for you," she said, with such positivity and love in her voice.

I looked in the mirror and saw my eyes that looked dull, haunted, heartbroken, exhausted, "Sure. Nice thought," I thought to myself. "but no happy endings here."

Sure enough, Leah was right: a happy ending did come in the form of my husband.

Dare I believe her again? I left the store holding the book tightly in my hands.

Tonight, I put the little photo album on my nightstand. I am so afraid I will lose it, and that will be a sign that my baby's picture will never be in it.

I check and recheck that the album is still there several times before letting myself fall asleep.

Leah and I have always been each other's cheerleaders when it comes to reaching our dreams. I believe she really does believe I'll have a baby. Just the way she believed I would find love again way back then.

What better gift can a friend give? Then to bestow upon another hope, a sense of believing that the one thing truly wished for will actually come true.

So I have this photo album, but I don't feel fully convinced that I will ever get to use it. I lift my head off the pillow, one more time, to make sure it is still on the nightstand before heading off to sleep.

In A Waiting Mode

Getting pregnant has overtaken my thoughts like never before.

When I started infertility treatments last year, I felt an easy confidence: of course I will get pregnant soon, I thought, I'm going to a clinic, taking medication, this is going to work out.

Now that time has passed and I'm still not pregnant, a lot of fear has set in. I worry pretty much all the time.

What if I'm one of those women for whom infertility treatments don't work? What if I try and try and never get pregnant?

My desire for a baby has reached a point where what I think about and talk about most of the time is having a child: will I have a child? Why am I not pregnant?

Thank God that at work, we are allowed to talk during the day. I work in member outreach at a PBS station in Boston, MA, where we call members for donations. It is a part-time job that allows me to get insurance for me and my husband, the pay isn't bad, and it isn't so stressful that it takes up all the time and space in my life. It is the perfect job for this time in my life right now.

The best part of the job are the wonderful people I have met, Judy and Chelsea. We all are very comfortable with one another, natural friends and we share a lot with each other. Judy has four children, and like myself, she cherishes children.

One day, out of the blue, Judy looked over at me and said, "I picture you with a daughter with corkscrew curly hair."

Hope! My dear friend was giving me hope! She was sharing with me a positive vision for my future! I can't thank Judy enough for gifting me with these words...words that I desperately need to hear. Hope is what I'm hanging on to by a thread right now...Hope...from a dear friend...much appreciated.

Shot Night

Tonight, for the first time, my husband administered the shots. All day long, I felt a heaviness hanging over me. At 2 p.m. it was five hours away. At 3 p.m. four hours away. At 4 p.m., three hours away.

Finally, it was 7 o'clock. My husband starts by opening the bottles to prepare the medication. I admire his bravery, as I watch him mix the medicines.

Then I sit down in the kitchen. I've learned a few tricks about taking tests:

1) Don't look. Keep your eyes shut. Seeing it only make the pain more intense.

2) Breath out, while blowing, blowing, blowing, kind of like as substitution.

3) Distract yourself with something fun, comforting or sweet.

4) Have a reward waiting.

Here's how I distracted myself tonight: I recently got a cookbook with recipes from bed and breakfast inns. The book has a beautiful blue and white cover and it is all about cozy, comfortable, romantic places..the delightful stuff bed & breakfast inns are made of.

I opened the book and decide that while I am getting a shot, I will read a recipe--knowing that by the time I get to the end of the recipe, the shot will be over.

We're just about ready. I am praying every moment for the strength to endure this. My husband looks for a spot on my leg. I look away.
I open to a recipe and start reading. The book is comforting and I am transported to a beautiful place.

My husband jabs the needle into my leg, quickly, so quickly, I breath, breath, breath. I pray. I start reading a recipe, and it is over. I've reached the end of my recipe.

Then, like a spring day after a storm, a bit of alcohol to clean it, a bandage and I am free. Tomorrow, I will think about the next shot. But for tonight, it is over and done. It hurt, but not half as bad as I imagined.

Now I can just sit back and enjoy tonight.

Another Shot Night

I'm getting more comfortable with the actual shots, although in the hours leading up to them, I am overcome with a lot of anxiety and dread.

Tonight, some of Chris's friends came over and we went ahead with the shots, despite the fact that they were all standing two feet away in our living room.

Having a bunch of guys standing outside the kitchen, practically watching me get shots, brought an air of humor to this. These guys are mostly single, so completely out-of-touch with this type of stuff, and so it was funny to see them privy to what is normally such an intimate and hush-hush procedure.

They actually seemed scared in a way, and that made the whole thing all the more humorous to me.

Friday Night Longing

It is a beautiful dark starry summer night and I feel anything but carefree.

Tomorrow I will go home to listen to my answering machine and find out the news. Bad news, I am pretty sure. The answer is going to be no. I know it. The answer for me is always no. I have learned that whenever I really want something, ultimately the answer always turns out to be no. I have come to understand that when I really want something, or someone, truly love this person, this thing, this whatever, the answer is no. So I already know the answer to the question I am waiting to hear answered. How else could it be?

I can barely stand to think of my future right now. It is Friday night and my cousin Susan has come to visit us. Susan is one of my favorite persons on this earth, and yet tonight, even her visit isn't cheering me up.
Susan had her children young in the most beautiful and normal way

people are suppose to have children. She is surrounded by children, grandchildren, and right now, in her presence, I feel woefully inadequate.

On my father's side of the family, it seems the tree bears fruit, in the normal way the cycle of life is suppose to work. Childbearing, getting pregnant, having children, comes easily, naturally, the family growing and multiplying. No one is alone or freakish. Life blossoms beautifully. They are part of the normal life continuum.

Susan doesn't know I'm going to an infertility clinic. She might vaguely suspect I want children, but she has no idea that tonight I feel like the biggest failure in the world in her presence. She was a grandmother at 36. Here I am, 33 years old and still no children. I once thought waiting until you were older to have children was the thing to do, and now I realize that the tables have turned and actually I am the unnatural freak who missed the biological boat.

Susan, my parents and myself go down to the center to get some fried dough and pizza. The "center" as we call this part of the beach is to an outsider nothing but a honky tonk bunch of neon signs, fried food, men in tattoos wearing leather jackets and girls with store bought bleached hair and too little clothes. But to my family, the center is a place of beautiful, never-to-be forgotten memories, of amusement park rides and favorite ice creams, the bright lights thrilling us in the darkness. It is the place where me and my cousins Sheri and Tina roamed around as teenagers, enjoying the tiny element of danger the night held, along with the ice cream and moon pies at Willy's, and most of all, the camaraderie of family. Usually, staying at my favorite beach in the world, one laden with such glorious childhood memories, and having my beloved cousin Susan sleep over, would feel like a great and grand treat. But tonight, the world feels ugly and sad to me. I am too old to be longing for the past. I should be over wanting and yearning for what used to be by now. Everywhere I look tonight, the past feels so much better than the present or even the future. It seems that at 12 years old, I had more than I have now--more connection, more family, more love, more fun. A child would bring it all back, change the life I have now.

 In the presence of my cousin who had four children by the time she was my age, I feel dull, barren, like a wrinkled fruit that never fully ripened. I live my life missing the past, and I'm tired of that...Tired of looking back all the time. I want a reason, a someone, to look forward for.

I need someone to create new memories for, rather than yearning for people and memories long gone in my life.

I want a child to introduce me to a new way of being, and reconnect with an old way of being that I have lost.

I want to be part of the club. That's it...I want to be a member in the natural process of life. I want to do what people, animals, bugs, birds, and all living beings have been doing since the earth came into existence.

Trees have leaves, squirrels have baby squirrels, from dirt comes weeds, plants and flowers, the sky gives out rain and ants breed more ants, and even old trees find a way to resurrect themselves in the spring to heave out a few more twigs and a few more leaves. Then, why is having a baby so hard for me?

Why, from the beginning, has everything about creating my own family been hard for me, from getting married to now having a baby? Why is this natural part of life such a struggle for me? My cousins seem to get married and have children without barely a thought, they so fit in the natural cycle of life, and yet for me, having my own family is a grueling, frustrating, nearly impossible dream.

I sat in the car while my parents and Susan went to get pizza at a place we've been going for years. I feel too sad to enjoy pizza or even get my body to move out of the car.

I stay in the car while they get in line for the pizza--I cannot bring myself to participate in the buzz of life going on around me tonight, when there is no buzz in my life that even remotely mirrors what is happening in the center tonight or what has happened here for generations.

I cannot help but thinking that by the time Susan was my age, she had given birth four times. I remember her at my age--she was all mother, all grown-up, a part of life's process. She had a family, a definite somewhere to belong in this world.

I sit in the car, watching all the life around me, the life I used to believe I would have long ago when I came here as a child. I feel like such a failure right now. The drizzle starts to fall and my heart is slowly and dully breaking.

News Arrives

Today I woke up with one thought in my mind: get out of here before you get the news. I'm am a raging volcano ready to explode.

If I call my house, check my answering machine, and hear' no, sorry-you-are-not-pregnant, I am going to flip out'. No, I am going to die. I am going to blame everyone around me for my life, for my lonely existence in a childless world. So this morning, I made some excuse about needing to go home to do some work on my online magazine, and I borrowed my mother's red Toyota Camry.

The drive home was fast, as I live only about 35 minutes from the beach. The Toyota ran so smoothly I felt like I was flying. I drive a clunky old Volvo, and I'm not used to this feeling of gliding down the highway. The ride home, so mockingly free, gave me a reprieve from my pain.

When I got home, I went straight up to our office where the answering machine lives. The red button was not blinking. I pressed play. Nothing. No message.

What happened is clear: my husband came home, played out the sad message of no, and decided not to save it, so as to spare me the pain. He wants to tell me himself.

He is right. I feel better not hearing it. I like the silence. I've heard enough no's loud and clear in my life. I don't want to hear no again. My husband is kind, and I feel a dull sense of relief, although I know this means terrible choices wait ahead for me.

We've done seven IUIs now, and I'm growing more convinced that the reason I can't get pregnant is that my eggs and my husband's sperm don't want to mate. What next? Look for somebody else's sperm? A pretty immoral idea, but not one I haven't toyed with.

My husband says fine, go do what you want, and a part of me screams yes, I deserve to be able to find a better biological choice, because above all else, I want children. Terrible. Horrible thoughts. I would never actually do something so immoral, but this is where sadness can lead: to desperate ideas that are wrong and that I would never do.

I get on my computer, one of the few places in this world where serenity comes over me.

I am working on my online magazine, and I have met an amazing web designer named Ann Sowers who is going to redesign the site.

When I'm working on Commitment, I become enraptured, in flow, and my thoughts of bearing children are replaced with creative thrill for a short time.

When I work on my magazine, I escape, if just for a few minutes, from being the washed out failure I am. I am dashing out West in my covered wagon, towards a new life.

Working on Commitment always calms me down. A few hours pass and it is almost time to get back to the beach.

I'm going to hear no tonight. Right out loud tonight I will hear no.

But at least it will be from my husband, and not from the voice of a nurse doing her routine calls, who says 'no, you are not pregnant' with the same kind of faux sympathy of a salesgirl who tells you, no, that blouse is no longer on sale, but try back next week.

I need to get back to the beach.

Part II: Secondary Infertility

Baby Making With Husband Nowhere In Sight

Today was my third IUI trying for a second child. Today was different than any of the other IUIs I've done before. My husband and I were not even together during the IUI. We went to the clinic at different times, in separate cars.

Because he had to work all day, and there was an ice cream festival at my work that my mother and I were bringing my daughter to, my husband drove to the clinic at 7 a.m., gave his sperm, and went off to work. An hour later, I arrived for my IUI.

How odd, I thought as I was driving to the clinic, I am now going to make a baby with my mother and my daughter, with my husband nowhere in sight. I felt sorry for myself, because as a young teenage girl, I would have never imagined that my baby making experience would include my mother, a nurse, and a speculum that really, really hurt.

Not that the other IUIs have ever felt natural to me, but having my husband at the clinic with me felt at least more normal--at least, I reasoned, we were doing this together.

Imagine how far science had come--that two people can make a baby separated by a few hours and several miles.

Nothing at all romantic about this baby-making exchange.

When I was young, and imagined having children, I never could have imagined that this would my future. Thank God I didn't know it would turn out this way. Thank God no one at 17 ever showed me a crystal ball into my baby-making future. My heart would have been broken. But I want another baby so much, that most of the time I dismiss these sentimental yearnings, I can't let anything interfere with my fertility treatments.

But today the yearnings got me good, and I feel a heavy load of melancholy.

I am so far away from the original way people usually create a family.

Once the IUI was over, my Mom and I drove to the ice cream festival at my workplace, a PBS station in Boston. Some of my co-workers got to meet my daughter for the first time.

As we drove home, my mother turned to me said, "Maybe you are pregnant."

Her hopefulness was sweet.

It must have been weird for my mother to go with me to the clinic, while I went into a room to be impregnated with my husband's sperm.

I can only imagine what my mother was thinking. But my Mom, always brave and tactful, didn't say anything mean or negative.

That night, I told my husband how sad I was that we were not together for today's IUI. He said he felt the same way.

 He doesn't take things as passionately as I do, or get as worked up when things don't work out. I think because I had such high expectations for love and romance, that times like this put a spotlight on how far I've travelled from the original dream for my life.

I have to let it go. I know I am so lucky to have my first baby. I could feel it today when I walked into that waiting room with my beautiful daughter and I saw the expressions on the faces of some of the women, and even men, when my daughter and I began to play with some toys. Their eyes lit up--a baby! Their eyes looked sad--a baby!...Someone else's as usual. I remember how I used to feel when someone would come into the waiting room with a baby. I felt excited, resentful, frustrated all at the same time. Sometimes seeing their success in having a baby made me hopeful. Sometimes their success made me jealous. Sometimes I felt all goopy to see a baby and to dare to imagine what it must feel like to have little hands to hold and cheeks to kiss.

I saw in the faces of the couples in the waiting room that same longing, mixed with hopefulness. So I know I shouldn't complain.

Tonight, I want to just snuggle up with my husband, and imagine that I am 17 and still allowed to believe that babies are made in bed by two people madly in love.

Oops! Pee Pee Problem

The hardest part of the IVF was something I did not expect at all.

It was not the myriad of shots I had to endure every night, or the insane number of times I had to drive Route 128 during the height of the morning commute.

It was having to hold my urine after the IVF. After the eggs and sperm were mixed together and planted back into me, I was wheeled back to the room and told to hold my urine for a half an hour.

I did not know that to help the eggs and sperm take hold, they have you drink an enormous glass of water and hold it.

This sounds simple, right?

Wrong.

It was hard.

So, so hard.

I laid there, dying to just get to a toilet and let it all flow out.

Holding one's pee pee has to be one of the hardest things to do on this earth.

Every part of me was screaming, "Let me go! Let me go! Let me go!"

Nothing in this whole process felt as horrible as being forced to hold an enormous amount of pee. I am expulsive by nature and inherently holding things in--feelings, anything--is grueling and painful.

"How many minutes?" I kept saying to my husband. I'd look at the clock. Five minutes had passed... I wanted to get up and disobey them, but I want this baby so bad...

I stared at the clock: one minute down, five minutes down..ten minutes down. It went so slow.

I hoped that by staring down the clock, the minutes would pass quicker.

Finally, I hit the thirty minute mark. I vaulted out of the bed into the bathroom.

Relief....it never felt so good.

Now I head home and wait for the results to find out if the IVF worked and I am pregnant.

Try, Try Again

I woke up the other morning and knew it had happened.

"I think I got it," I whispered to my husband.

"Oh no," he said softly, in a heavy tone full of sadness.

I tip-toed quietly to the bathroom.

"Yes," I confirmed a few minutes later. "I got it."

The red hot signal that I am not pregnant had arrived.

Inside me, walls came crashing down and others went up.

I should be pregnant. I should be, should
be, should be!

"We'll keep trying for a baby," my husband said kindly.

Try? How dare he! Try was not a word I wanted to hear. The very word 'try' enraged me. Try? Trying isn't an option....we'll make this happen! We'll will it to happen, force it to happen, bend its arm backwards and make it happen.

"What do you mean 'trying'?" I asked him, frustrated that he would relegate having our second child to simply an act of trying and not an act of will.

"I said we'll keep trying," he repeated, not at all understanding why I was getting so mad at him.

The rest of the day was a fuzzy blur. I ended up with a razor sharp headache and a stomache. The next day, I find out that two of my friends are pregnant. They are certainly not specimens of health and yet they are pregnant.

Why is it so easy for some people? Why is it so hard for me?

I need a plan and came up with this:

• My husband will see a nutritionist to strengthen and improve his sperm.

• I will see the same nutritionist.

• I will also go to a person who specializes in emotional release. Sounds flaky, I know, but a friend highly recommends it and for $35 I figure why not try it.

The premise is that trapped emotion in the body can cause illness and dysfunction, and that once negative emotion is released, the body can return to health and normalcy.

My guess is that deep inside me, some sadness is trapped, and perhaps it needs to be released in order for everything in my body to work properly--kind of like an old clock with a big piece of dust preventing the hands from turning.

• I will go to acupuncture once, sometimes twice, a week.

• I will begin eating an extremely healthy diet. I started eating healthier a few months ago, and recently I have seen a big increase in the number of eggs I am producing.

• I will also swim everyday, or every other day. Swimming for me is a great stress reliever.

• I will pray more, although I already pray about 1,000 times a day. Prayer is a privilege that I cannot imagine living without. Thank God that He gave us the ability to talk to Him and go to Him for help. I will ask God to show me what I need to do in order to heal my body and conceive a second child.

Writing My Life Story and Seeing Patterns

Next week is my appointment with Begbetti, a homeopathic expert in Cambridge, MA.

She mailed me a questionnaire and asked me to write my life story, that will help her determine what patterns in my life need to be unblocked.

Writing this life story has been revealing. It seems my life has two themes running simultaneously: one is about joy, happiness, friendship, achievement and faith. The other theme is loss and rejection.

I wrote about losing my best friend in seventh grade to the 'cool kids' and this pattern of loss, followed by great mourning and sadness, seems to be a reoccurring theme in my life.

There seems to be a lot of dramatic endings in my relationships. It was hard to write this and see in black-and-white all my failures.

I'm bringing a copy of my life story to Eileen so she can work on helping me to release some these memories. I know all these painful losses live inside me and are sapping physical strength from me.

How can I successfully carry a baby for nine months, when I carry around so many lost people in my heart?

Praying Hard

Prayer is an integral part of my infertility treatments. God is my partner in this infertility quest.

I don't pray expecting that if I make all the wrong choices, I'll still get a baby. I pray that He gives me the strength to keep trying when I want to give up. I pray that He helps me find the right doctors and do the right things to heal my body.

I don't naively think if I pray for a baby, but drink sugary soda, miss important appointments, keep on this extra weight, and guzzle coffee that my body is going to produce the baby of my dreams.
I know God hears my prayers and I know He wants good things for me, but I also believe He has gifted me with power over my life to some degree. I have the power to make choices, to investigate information and pursue treatments that will help me.

So I don't just pray to have a baby, but I also pray to find the right treatments to heal my infertility.

I read that when you have a goal, you have to be ready to walk through fire to attain the goal.

Well, I'm ready. I would cut off my foot if it guaranteed that I would have a baby. I will go anywhere, spend any amount of money I have, try just about anything to make my body able to conceive and give birth.

I have to work along with my prayers, and if my prayer is for a baby, I have to be doing things to get myself healthy enough to have a baby.

I think the biggest lie told about God is that He wants to deny humans and say no to their requests whenever possible.

I can't say how many people have said right out loud, or insinuated, that God may not want me to have a second baby. Why do so many people naturally and easily assume that if I want a second baby, God doesn't want me to have one? Why do they find it so easy to think God wants to deny me what I most want? Why can't they think that God wants good things for me--and why wouldn't a second baby be good for me?

Why is everyone so ready to attribute everything bad or denied in their life to God saying no, when really it could be their own choices, their own lack of initiative and willpower, or their own choice to stay a victim rather than work hard to improve the situation?

If I give up now, should I blame God if I never have a second child--or blame myself for giving up?

Maybe God wants me to have a baby, but He is leaving it up to me to keep trying. I do not blame God for my infertility. I blame human imperfection. I am sick. I am not ashamed that I have infertility problems. I am tired of people insinuating there is something shameful about my condition.

I am not ashamed.

I am not a bad person because I have problems getting pregnant.

I am not a weak person, a morally bad person, a cursed person, or a woman punished by God.

I am not weird and do not deserved to be whispered about because of my problem.

I am a person with a health problem, who is seeking to get healthier and who is asking God to help me.

I do not pray and eat Twinkies. I do not pray and do nothing. That would be an insult to the power God has given me over my life.

I have choices. I have the ability to seek out answers to the questions in my life, and right now, the question is: why is my body having trouble getting pregnant?

I think God wants me to have another baby. I think He wants my daughter to have a sibling to love. I think He will help me.
I think He also expects me to work hard for this myself. I do not assume He will say no just because I want to hear a yes.

Does Loss of Authentic Personality Equals Loss of Fertility?

 Today was my first appointment with Dr. Zhu, an acupuncturist and master herbalist, who I wanted to try because I've heard a lot of wonderful things about Chinese herbs helping infertility.

 I have to say that driving to his office was among the worst driving experiences I've had lately. But then, driving to the clinic is pretty harrowing too.

I have no choice but to drive this highway, but sometimes I feel like the drive down Route 128 is a metaphor for my infertility: you must do what you have to do to get to your destination, regardless of how frightening and horrifying it feels.

Dr. Zhu's office was so peaceful, in contrast to my drive over. He felt my pulse, which acupuncturists and Chinese herbalists do to determine what is wrong. He then had me read a paragraph from a book on what he considered to be some of my problems. The paragraph described me perfectly.

Then he put together a bag of herbs for me to boil and make into a tea.

Before I left, he gave me a short, but very powerful, acupuncture treatment. During Dr. Khu's treatment, I could actually feel parts of my brain opening that had been closed off for a long time.

After he inserted the needles, I sat reading a 'People' magazine article about the problem of bullying in the school systems, and how one young boy even committed suicide because he was so tormented by bullies.
I was overwhelmed with inspiration, got out my notebook and started

jotting down ideas how to curb the bullying problem.

In all, I wrote nine pages on how to stop bullying and while I wrote, I felt different than I had in a long time: powerful and capable of changing things, unblocked by the usual shame, fear, embarrassment or failure I often feel when I imagine that I can change things. It was like an old part of me resurfaced that wasn't ashamed or burdened down with memories of failures.

Charging forward with solutions and fighting for causes was a part of who I was long time ago. Over time, and with lots of failures, I lost this part of me who believed I could change things or make things better for others.

When I was a child, I was always coming up with ideas to fix things and right wrongs. I ran a Jerry Lewis carnival for muscular dystrophy, got signatures for a Save the Whales petition, and in college organized a two-week Feed the World weeks festival, where the governor of Massachusetts declared April 25 Feed the World Day.

'Feed the World' weeks turned out to be a big disaster. I was 19 and not really ready to undertake a fundraising operation of this size. We raised $5,000, but I made a million mistakes. The experience shrank me. After that, I never had the confidence to spearhead anything again. When I heard about this crisis or that crisis, I no longer imagined that I could do something about it.

Maybe I lost the belief that I was competent enough to make positive change. I never consciously realized, or even acknowledged, that this change had come over me, but my life slowly became more about protecting, hiding and defending myself, rather than reaching out to help and make a difference.

Yet, all of a sudden during this treatment, I felt that activist part of me come back to life. I felt angrily energized about the problem of bullying in America and I somehow felt capable of coming up with solutions to the problem, much the way I used to feel when I was young.

Is it possible that this acupuncture treatment resurrected a dead part of me that was once a pillar of my personality? And how did losing this part of me relate to my infertility?

Is my infertility related to an inability to manifest my will and power in this world?

What is the correlation between my infertility and this loss in my personality?

I can't speculate too much about this--as I don't really know what this treatment did to me exactly, but I wonder if the disappearance of who I am also weakened my body's ability to manifest things I care about in general.

I left very contented to have added yet another layer to my healing.

My Most Private Journals: What My Subconscious Had To Say
Here's a peek at the journals I wrote from the point of view of my subconscious as I tried to dig out what my subconscious self was truly feeling and experiencing at this time.

Journal 1

Me: I am having a baby.

Subconscious: A baby--you? You big loser? You know what a loser you are. A baby? You couldn't have a pet cat if you tried. (Note: today I have four pets cats so I guess my subconscious was very wrong!) A baby--oh my God, everyone knows you are too old and too worn out. You can't handle anything. Do you realize what a screw up you are? Paula, the road to hell is paved with good intentions, and you are that road to hell. I can't believe you think this can work out. Get a grip.

Me: I am having a baby. I am having a healthy beautiful baby. I am pregnant right now.

Subconscious: Oh God, you are nothing. I can't believe you buy this optimism crap. I think you better give up my dear, because you are worthless.

Me: My vagina is strong and my baby is growing healthy inside me. I can carry a baby.

Subconscious: You can't carry a baby. Hasn't it been proven your eggs are too old and too messed up? You have some problem--maybe mercury, but give up weirdo. You are indeed a big weirdo. You are not like all the other women who had babies young. You are too old. You are very old.

Me: I am pregnant and in nine months I'm going to have a baby.

Subconscious: Wishful thinking. You are meant to struggle and get nothing. You are meant to be perpetually punished for your sins. No one ever believes in you.

Me: I like myself. I believe I can have more babies. I am strong. I make good eggs.

Subconscious: Stop the bravado. It isn't working on me. I feel like you can't have any more kids. Dr. M said you were too old--and I believe her. You look old. You feel old. You seem like the world has gone by you on this one. God hates you too. How could He like you? How in the world could you think God would help you?

Me: I can have babies. I am having more babies. My body is creating more babies.

Subconscious: Your friend had a baby with one ovary, barely made any eggs, and somehow got a baby out of the deal, a nice boy baby. You are not looking for gold--you want one more baby. You can do this. Look, it may be hard. It may be a long road. No one said this will be easy. You need help along the way. But ultimately, you can have a baby. You won't do stupid things. You'll rest a lot. You'll go to Eileen and Dr. Deutsch a lot. You'll get help.

Journal 2: I ask my body why it was having trouble getting pregnant.

Me: Why can't I have a baby?

Subconscious: Because you are bad. Because you are not worth anything. Because you get envious and anxious and something is wrong with you. Because you are not worth anything. Because you deserve nothing

Me: Why can't I have another baby?

Subconscious: Because you only get one shot at happiness. Because you can't escape your fate.
Me: I hate my life. I am stuck. I am in a hole. I am disappearing. I'm tired of people telling me to give up and accept. I am never giving up! That is not me. I am not giving up at all. I never give up when I want something. I want a second baby. No! I want ten babies. Two is not enough. I want many, many, many, babies. Give me more babies! Give me more!

Subconscious: No! You are a bad girl. Other girls will get everything-- you get nothing. You are a loser. You can't escape your life. You are a weirdo. A loser.

The Second IVF Begins Now

 I am entering a climatic, exciting, and frantic zone.

So much build-up...now reaching a crescendo.

I went this morning for a blood test and I found out that Sunday will be the day of my egg retrieval, Wednesday the implantation, and it all starts tonight with my HCG shot between 7 and 8 p.m.

 I've waited since last February for this moment—and it ends up happening on the same weekend as Leah's going away party and my cousin Lori's wedding.

Because the shot needs to be taken by 8 p.m. tonight, I can only stay an hour at Leah's going away party. That is how infertility is--it butts into your life and demands priority regardless of what else is going on.

I built this party up so much to my daughter, talked on and on about "the fun we were going to have at Aunt Leah's party" and now we will basically walk in to the party, say hi, give a few hugs and leave.

I could easily start screaming.

Why is this happening at the same time I have to say goodbye to one the most important people in my life?

A part of me wants to hide out until my baby is born and not deal with anything but baby making. God, I have to get pregnant soon. How many more IVFs will they let me do? How many chances do I get? I can't delve into that murky place right now. This time has got to work.

After all this waiting, it boils down to now. Tonight, finally.

Leah will leave for Portland in a few days. I won't see her after the party tonight. She has been there beside me through everything the past 10 years. How am I going to do without her?

The pain of her leaving is starting to make me physically ache. I can't focus on this or I will fall apart.

I've waited so long for this IVF and now finally it is here. I think I am ready.. I just didn't think it would all start tonight.

We were one of the first ones to arrive at Leah's going away party. I couldn't really explain to her mother why we couldn't stay long. As usual, I feel like I am walking around keeping secrets. Ssh--don't tell anyone. I'm taking my shot tonight. Always, always secrets. Then tomorrow is my cousin's wedding. Chris is stressing about money again because I'm going to see Eileen on Tuesday so she can prepare my body for the implantation Wednesday. Between her and Dr. Deutsch, it will cost about $140. Chris is cranky about this, but I told him I need to go. Good God, to come so far and not do everything possible to make this happen--that would be crazy.

I'm trying not to show Leah how sad I am right now and I'm trying to tell myself that we will always stay close and in touch.
My gut tells me that she will return, but another part of me wonders: will she end up living across the country for the next 20 years? Is one of the most important persons in my life permanently leaving.

I made an attempt to act brave and casual with Leah, talking excitedly about Portland and the wonderful people she is going to meet. I told her how proud I was of her for making this daring move.

I am just feeling very sad for myself.

Around 6:45 p.m., we say goodbye. I feel selfish leaving the party so early, but the shot has to be priority right now. Leah and I stood at the door of the old Grange hall, hugging tightly. Leah starts to cry, and I am just about overwhelmed by a tidal wave of grief. I try to hold it back. I can't let myself despair over her departure. She is doing what she needs to do to create the life she wants, and I am doing what I need to do to create the life I want.

Oh, if only it was all so cut and dry. My dear beloved, best friend Leah is leaving!

We got home, and at exactly 8 o'clock, Chris gave me the shot. Now, my ovaries are cooking with eggs. Oh God, please let me get pregnant. Please God, make this work. I've done so much, prepared and waited so long, please God don't let me be disappointed.

To read the entire The Infertility Diaries are available on Amazon.com or at www.dancingyourwaytofertility.com.

News

Today was my pregnancy test. I think I know the answer.

The nurse's called later that day: No, I'm not pregnant. I did, however, have a chemical pregnancy however and it did not continue. The words shake me to the core. What is this thing called chemical pregnancy?

Tell me everything, explain this to me, I ask. Why did this happen? Was it my eggs? Is it because of the quality of my eggs?

I am not trying to be a pain, but I need answers.

The nurse is annoyed. She barely answers my questions.

No, I am not crazy. I just want an explanation.

The nurse is cold, aloof, off-putting. As if I have no right to ask so many questions.

I dial the clinic again and get the voice mail for my nursing team. I leave a question.

A few minutes later, I call again. I leave another question. I call again 12 minutes later. I have more questions. I can't stop calling. I can't stop asking questions. I need answers. No one is giving me answers. No one is explaining why this happened. I dial again, and leave more questions. I need to know. Am I on the wrong medication?

What is going on with me? I need information. If only I could understand this. Why isn't anyone telling me anything?

One nurse in particular is extremely rude to me. She acts as if I'm complaining about an order gone wrong at a drive through. She doesn't have time for me and I know she thinks I'm crazy. Maybe I am crazy. Yes, I am crazy today. Who can blame me? Who can blame me for being crazy? What am I suppose to be--rational after all this?

I dial again and leave more questions. I can't stop even though I know I should. No one is answering me! No one is helping me! I feel compelled to act. Give me answers! Give me information! Please, tell me right now what went wrong and why.

Finally, a kind nurse calls me back. Her name is Chris and she is very sympathetic. She tries to answer my questions, but she doesn't have the answers.

I ask her if she thinks I'll ever get pregnant again. She tries to sound hopeful, without giving me false hope that could make the clinic liable. I appreciate her kindness and trying to answer my questions the best she could. She is so different from the other nurses.

I will never forget the kindness of this nurse who called me back.

I have so many questions. I need to make an appointment with my doctor to discuss everything about my treatment, from the amount of progesterone I am given, to my medication. Something is wrong.
I can't believe this is happening!
I feel a crazy inconsolable kind of anger and helplessness.

A few minutes later, a counselor from the clinic calls to see how I am doing. Probably that mean nurse reported me, told the counselor to call the crazy woman leaving too many messages on the voice mail. I quickly get a grip and feign saneness while I talk to her. I'm frightened she will report that I am too nuts to go through another IVF.

I hate this counselor. She has to be the most insensitive, cruel counselor imaginable. She tells me some awful statistic on women my age getting pregnant. She goes on to list all the problems that can be expected at my age. Is that what she thinks is going to comfort me? What a freakin' idiot! I wish I could report her to someone, but if I do, she will label me as psychotic and they will kick me out of the clinic.

Someday I'll write a letter to the clinic telling them about the complete insensitivity of this supposed counselor.

I wonder how many other woman she made feel hopless during their darkest moments. She has no right to hold this position, but I need to stay quiet right now and pretend I am okay.

I tell her I feel fine. Yes, I am disappointed, I say casually, but I'll get over it. She seems to accept that. The idiot can be tricked so easily. I thank her for calling. She asks if I want an appointment, and instead of saying no, I tell her I have my daughter to care for and getting a sitter is hard, but yes, eventually I would love to come in for an appointment.

What a stupid lady. She falls for it, hook, line and sinker. I hate playing this game with her, but she scares me.

She is mean enough and lacks insight in such full measure that if I tick her off in any way, she will say I'm not psychologically fit to handle another IVF. So I pull myself together during this phone call and I act like I'm fine and okay about this pregnancy gone wrong, not a woman with any emotion, thank you.

My husband seems confused too. Has the possibility of having another baby already escaped us? I go crazy at the thought.
I have a million questions and no answers. This was not at all what I expected.

Chemical Pregnancy Nightmare

Why didn't I get pregnant this time?

No one seems to be able to tell me why.

I have an appointment to talk with my doctor. I mailed her a letter with 20 questions, so that she can take some time and review my particular case before we meet.

Am I on the right medicine? Am I getting enough progesterone? Do I need some type of test to determine whether there is a virus in my body causing these problems? And if so, do I need a strong and swift antibiotic to be rid of this infection?

I hope sending the questions ahead of time will make it possible for her to thoroughly research all my questions.

I want everyone to just go away and leave me alone.

Devastating Meeting

Today was my meeting with Dr. N. I woke up excited. Finally! I'll get some answers! She has my questions and had lots of time to research them.

I have been reading about some new medications, and there are some medicines out there that seem to suit me. I am requesting a change.

I wore my red suit, with the idea that maybe, if I looked professional, she would take me seriously. Boy, was I in for a surprise.

Instead of going over the questions, she immediately began talking about the number of messages I left on the nursing team's voice mail. She alluded to the fact that her nurses were aggravated with me.

Immediately, I knew this meeting wasn't going in a good direction.

I'm being tested right now, I thought, and I better remain cool if I ever want the chance to do another IVF at this clinic again.

I immediately apologized for my persistent phone calls, and explained that a first, I was very upset.

Then she asked if I was okay now, and if I felt I was able to take doing another IVF.

"I'm fine," I smiled convincingly "I was upset, but I'm over it. I understand these things happen."

Hah! I really wanted to say: Doctor, I'm still a basket case, but obviously, you, like everyone else around here, wants me to feel no emotion at all. You prefer me to be just another quiet little number in the pecking order. Take my disappointment and shove it down. Ask no questions. Make no demands. Make no waves. Exactly what everyone wants out of women everywhere--to stay silent and just be good little soldiers who do as they are told without ever protesting or questioning or feeling.

That's right ladies, you should feel nothing regardless of what you are going through. Say nothing, accept whatever is handed to you without any emotion at all. And you, being a women doctor, should know better, teach your nurses better, understand more. I expected more from you, but you are no different than the people who have wanted to silence women for years. I get it.

I'm too much work, too much hassle, and you have no time to answer 22 questions. I understand the rules here: passion, sadness, hysteria, desperation, is in no way allowed. I understand. I am suppose to do this without feeling.

I'm suppose to take the bad news and cry silently alone, and never bother anyone with my pain.

Then she went on to suggest that maybe I take some test to determine my ovarian reserve and chances of getting pregnant. No way, I think, I am not taking some test so you can label me unable to conceive and then insurance will stop all my treatment.

I tell her maybe later, it sounds good, but I want to do another IVF first.

She looks at me quite seriously and tells me that because of the amount of medication I need, it looks as if my eggs are at the bottom of the barrel.

Everything stops for a minute. The little trickle of hope I had left oozes away. I didn't expect this.

She says for my age, I need way too much medication. She questions if I ever smoked, and I tell her I never even tried a cigarette in my life. She seems to not believe me, and asks again. I repeat that I've never even tried a cigarette in my life. She now recommends that I look into donor eggs, and I think: no, I'm not doing that.

Then I tell her that despite all my problems, I think I still have a chance of having one more child. "All I need is for one egg to turn out right," I say, trying to sound reasonable, logical, defending myself against her attack, but most of all fighting the hopelessness building inside me.

"Maybe," she says, with an expression that means "keep dreaming dummy."I ask her if she wants to go over any of my questions. She glances quickly at them. It is obvious she hasn't gone over them. She says they don't apply.

I ask about changing my medication. She doesn't want to consider it right now.

I rise to leave. We shake hands and I pretend I am okay.

I thank her for her time.

Once I get in the car, I feel wildly, frantically angry. I am stunned. I can't even cry. I drive home in a daze. Her words ring in my head: your eggs are the bottom of the barrel. Your eggs are bottom of the barrel...your eggs are bottom of the barrel."

 I never realized it was this bad. Regardless of everything I've gone through, I never felt like my time was up.

My time can't be up! I need another baby--I need a baby for my daughter! I can't accept this...I can't live with this.

I start to pray. I pray and I pray and I pray, because I know under no uncertain terms that it will only be through God's help that I will ever get a baby now.

I am at such a desperate point. Her words have nearly broken my will and spirit. Thank God I know God. Thank God I can pray to God. If I didn't have God and His gift of prayer, I would give up right now.

After I pray, for some reason I can't explain, I stop on the way home at a big alternative supermarket in my area and go directly to their book section.

I am searching for hope.

I start reading a book on women's health written by Christine Northrup, *Women's Bodies, Women's Wisdom* and I come upon her chapter on reproduction and fertility.

She writes that in other cultures, it is perfectly normal for women in their late 40s to have babies. She thinks that some of the infertility problems in the United States are because women are told they are too old to have babies in their 30s. This is wrong, she says, and the problems stem primarily from lifestyle, eating habits and stress.

A little bit of hope returns, and I thank God for physicians like Dr, Northrup who give women hope, instead of ripping it away like Dr. M.

I had switched to Dr. M I assumed that because she was a woman, she would have more empathy and more of a bedside manner than Dr. S., but I was wrong.

First, she misdiagnosed me with a fibroid and now she calls my eggs bottom of the barrel.

She obviously doesn't like to be hassled or bothered, and someone like me, who asked too much of her nursing team and mailed her 22 questions, was obviously too much work.

When I got home, a neighbor who had undergone infertility treatments was visiting. She recommended I switch to her doctor, who was in the same clinic.

I went upstairs to call my mother. I desperately needed to talk to my mother. It is times like these that it is my mother's voice I need to hear above all others.

There are few people on this earth who you can always count on to provide you with hope, but I am fortunate enough to say regardless of whatever has happened in my life, my mother has always given me hope.
My brilliant mother always understands that bottom line: hope will get

a person through. If she didn't do this, I don't know if I would have ever gotten past some of the disappointments in my life.

My mother is also very intelligent. She gave me this brilliant advice, "That doctor doesn't believe you can have a baby. I know you can. Change doctors. Do it today, immediately. If she is telling you this stuff, go to another doctor who is willing to work with you."

My mother was right. Why was I giving her opinion of my fertility so much power? My mother is right—let me see what another doctor has to say. I hung up with my mother, and immediately phoned the clinic to have my records transferred to Dr. G, my neighbor's doctor.

I set up an appointment for next week and mailed him the same 22 questions I had given Dr. M.

Dr. M has no idea what she did to me. If not for God and my mother, I might just give up on ever having another biological child. What kind of monster is she? Who is this doctor that thinks it is okay to rip a person's heart out? Maybe in her mind, she really thinks there is no hope for me.

Maybe she thinks I'm so crazy, that it is better to remove all hope from me.

Well, maybe I am a bit crazy, but I'm not so crazy as to stop trying.

She took some of the fight out of me today. I went there looking for answers and instead I got put in my place. A demanding, out-of-control, strong-willed woman being put in her place, ironically, by another woman. Not at all what I expected when I chose this doctor.

Tonight, in bed, anger and rage came over me. I wanted to phone the clinic and leave 100 nasty messages about this doctor and her cowardly nursing team.

My husband stopped me. "Give me the phone," I cried. "They all deserve to be told off! She deserves me to tell her what I think of her!"

"No, don't blow it," he warned.

"I don't want to ever go back to that clinic. I want to go to another clinic. She deserves to be told off," I say.

"Don't do it. If you do, you can't go back there. Just do another IVF and see what happens," he says reasonably.

"I can't stand it. I have to tell her off," I cry.

"Paula, don't blow this. If you tell them off, they will think you are crazy and they won't let you do another IVF. Not there, and maybe nowhere else either. Just do the IVF and maybe you'll get a baby next time," he says this with such reassurance that I calm down.

"You are right," I said. "But when I have my next baby, I am going to march into her office and say, "SEE YOU JERK! SEE THIS BEAUTIFUL BABY! THIS IS WHAT BOTTOM OF THE BARREL LOOKS LIKE!!!"

Bonus Excerpt from Dancing Your Way to Fertility available on

Amazon.com and at www.dancingyourwaytofertility.com.

Infertility: A Training Ground for Motherhood?

In times past, women have always endured sacrifice and trial as part of motherhood. Now, due to a host of factors such as age, health and environment, women are put through a severe test of their maternal stamina even before they conceive their child.

This road, this test, this initiation, will test all of you--and it will make you one of the strongest, most capable, confident, resourceful, perseverant mothers a child could ever have. Experiencing infertility gives you a lifetime pass to enjoy motherhood in a way few ever get to enjoy it, because with the difficulties of this disease come confidence and appreciation.

This journey will demand all the best parts of you. It will demand you persevere when you want to give up.

It will demand patience and persistence when frustration and helpless surrender might feel like a more natural path.
It will demand that every survival skill you possess be brought forth and utilized. It will demand sacrifice, self-preservation, and a willpower beyond what you knew you had, but what intrinsically you knew you were capable of.

If you are not fortunate, you may have your heart broken in 1000 pieces.

If you are fortunate, you could still have your heart broken in 1000 places.

When you give birth to your baby none of it will matter. Your heart will heal, the scars will seem insignificant, and all the tears, disappointments and devastations will seem like bunny rabbits and balloons on a summer's day.

No big deal.

If you do not give birth to a baby, but decide to adopt, become a foster parent, a teacher, coach, counselor or play a very active role in the life of a young niece, nephew, neighbor, or cousin, you will be ready and able to mother these children and impact a younger generation in a way more powerful than you ever imagined.

You have probably been through the best training course for motherhood possible: you understand pain, you understand the potential for joy, you are willing to do the work to get the child you want, and you've proven you can take the bad stuff that comes with going after the good stuff. In doing this, you will join a group of super cultivated mothers, women ready to nurture and love the next generation, and have more than proven their worth to do this.

Infertility hurts.

Winning over infertility can be a painful process that demands resolve and sacrifice.

It is an initiation rite, of sorts, an involuntary one, of course.

No one should have to go through this to have a baby and no one would voluntarily choose this road. Nonetheless, it is a reality for many of us, and it will prepare you for motherhood in a grand and inspiring way that someday you may even feel thankful to have experienced.

It is a long road and an unfair one, but at the end of the road, you could be holding the baby of your dreams, just as the same as someone who made love one night and woke up pregnant the next morning.

Then nothing at all will matter but your baby.

12 Cleanses To Help Restore Your Fertility

A Bonus Excerpt from Dancing Your Way to Fertility available on Amazon.com and at www.dancingyourwaytofertility.com.

The next step in changing the state, or condition, of your body is cleansing and detoxifying. The importance of detoxifying your body should never be underestimated. In this chapter, we'll look at 12 cleanses that can help restore and maximize your fertility potential.

Please note: cleanses should be done before you start infertility medications or treatments, because you do not want them to interfere with medications or a pregnancy, if there is even a slight chance you could be pregnant. Cleansing can be compared to overturning and fertilizing the soil before planting the seed.

If you are just starting infertility treatments, you may want to choose just one or two cleanses, so as not to delay treatment.

If you've been trying to get pregnant for a long time with no success, you might want to consider doing various cleanses to strengthen your body.
Here are some cleanses to consider:

• A Liver Cleanse

Never never NEVER underestimate the importance of having your liver cleaned and detoxified. The liver is a highly influential organ that plays a key role in fertility and is one of the most important organs in your body.

The liver governs approximately 500 metabolic processes and many studies have shown that the oestrogen receptors in the liver are critical for maintaining fertility.

I cannot say enough about the importance of having a clean, de-toxified liver in the quest to get pregnant.

An ineffective liver allows toxins to seep into the ovaries and endocrine system.

If your liver is congested, it cannot adequately remove toxins and fats from the body.

Instead, they will continue to recirculate through your system—causing hormonal disturbances and imbalances. It also means your ovaries will be flooded with toxic substances that your liver was suppose to clean— and your ovaries are the source of your eggs. These impurities will result in poor egg quality—all because your liver was too congested to do its job. So if you want to improve the quality of your eggs, make sure your liver is as clean and detoxified as possible.

Once the liver is cleansed, the entire endocrine and reproductive system becomes free of toxins and impurities, so they can begin functioning at a higher capacity.

What causes a sluggish, tired liver? Stress, poor diet, medication, toxins in the environment, low-quality food, coffee, sugar, white flour products and low quality drinking water, are among a few of the culprits. The older we get, the more our liver needs to be cleaned out because of the junk that we have taken into our body over the years.

A liver cleanse will help kick your body into high gear, increasing energy and vitality to all your organs.

Liver cleanses can be found online and at most health and natural food stores.

You may want to do a 30-day cleanse more than once. Please note: A liver cleanse should never be done while you are taking infertility medications, as it could interfere with the effectiveness of the medication. It is something to do BEFORE you begin any infertility treatments or medication, and is never to be done if you could be pregnant.

In addition to a liver cleanse, here are some other ways to detoxify, cleanse and strengthen your liver:

• Milk thistle is a wonderful herb for cleansing the liver. Read the directions on the bottle carefully as to amounts taken.

• Lemon is a great liver cleanser. About 20 minutes before breakfast in the morning, squeeze the juice from one or two fresh lemons into some warm water and drink.

• Beets are excellent liver cleansers. You can eat them cooked or juice them. To juice beets, peel and cut into small wedges that can easily fit in your juicer. Juice the beets with some apple, spinach or kale.

• Chlorophyll is a highly esteemed liver cleanser.

• Artichokes are powerful liver protectors because they contain a flavonoid called silymarin, which is an antioxidant that protects the liver from toxicity.

• Foods that are good for your liver include: spirulina, garlic, carrots, romaine lettuce, apples, grapefruit, chicory, mustard greens, dandelion greens, avocados, walnuts, turmeric and parsley.

• Cabbage can also be juiced and is effective in cleaning the liver.

• Amino acids, derived from healthy sources of protein, are key to the liver working at maximum capacity. Foods that contain these amino acids include: nuts, such as pumpkin seeds, squash seeds and almonds; lean meats, eggs, and beans, such as lentils and garbanzo.

• In Chinese medicine, infertility is often linked to Liver chi stagnation, a result of stress, overwork, and the effects of coffee and alcohol. Irritability, headaches and frustration are just some of the physical and emotional symptoms of liver chi stagnation. Acupuncturists and herbalists can work on unblocking energy stagnation in the liver.

• According to Chinese medicine, emotional and lifestyle cures for liver stagnation include being assertive, making clear decisions and enjoying lots of fun, laughter and relaxation. Holding on to anger, feeling stuck and depression impair the liver by stagnating the energy. Letting go, moving on, and exercising control over one's life, can help in healing the liver.

For more cleanses, visit DancingYourWayToFertility.com or Amazon.com.

How to Improve Your Egg Quality

A Bonus Excerpt from Dancing Your Way to Fertility available on Amazon.com and at www.dancingyourwaytofertility.com.

Good news—you can improve the health and quality of your eggs.

In the past, we were told we were all born with a certain number of egg cells that run out as we age. We were led to believe that egg cells were the only cells in the body that did not regenerate, but instead were a finite number. We are finding out THIS IS JUST NOT TRUE. Recent research has shown that women can produce new eggs throughout their reproductive years.

You may have been told that your eggs are not healthy or that your eggs are too old.

Here's the great news: there is much you can do to enhance the health of your eggs.

It was commonly believed that the only factor that determined egg health and quality was age. Several new studies have shown that stress, hormones and environmental toxins all impact our egg health.

Your egg's health is a key cornerstone of a healthy fertility, because the health of your eggs can affect whether or not fertilization, implantation and ultimately a healthy pregnancy and birth will occur.

Here are some things you can do to improve your egg health:

• Coenzyme Q10: Coenzyme Q10 is an excellent way to improve the quality and energy within your eggs.

In several studies, the supplement Coenzyme Q10 has been shown to improve egg quality.

It boosts energy production in the oocytes, which are cells in the ovary. Providing additional energy in the form of Coenzyme Q10 is needed when there is decreased energy production in the ovaries due to aging.

It is also a source of fuel for the mitochondria, which produces energy within the cells and with age, can begin to weaken. Along with taking a Coenzyme Q10 supplement, natural sources of CoQ10 include almonds, spinach, sardines, broccoli, strawberries, and walnuts.

For more on egg health, Dancing Your Way to Fertility is available on Amazon.com or visit www.dancingyourwaytofertility.com.

The People In Your Journey and Some of the Rude Comments You May Hear Along the Way

A Bonus Excerpt from Dancing Your Way to Fertility available on Amazon.com and at www.dancingyourwaytofertility.com.

This is not to be misinterpreted as an exercise in dumping family or friends, because people are not perfect and we should not expect them to be, and there are people in our lives, as unpleasant as they may be, that we simply need to forgive, stay connected to and be around.

Despite their flaws, we owe them something. That being said, as you walk this journey, you need to be ready for some of the stupid, rude and totally insensitive comments you are going to hear. Sometimes, people you love will say really dumb things.

Other times, it could be a stranger who zaps you with a statement that leaves you breathless and feeling punched in the gut.

Here are a few of the stupid, rude, thoughtless and COMPLETELY FALSE comments you may have to deal with, and how best to respond:

• "**Maybe you weren't meant to have a baby**": Yes, you were meant to have a baby. Yes, you were.

Millions of women have babies whether they want them or not, whether they will be good mothers or not, so why shouldn't you have a baby? In fact, there is NOT ONE REASON IN THIS UNIVERSE why you should not have a baby.

This person is either jealous of you or just likes to pop the balloon of hope. People who mouth off a comment like this mistakenly feel they have some sort of moral authority. Ignore them. They are wrong. Completely and utterly wrong.

• **"Aren't you a little too old to be trying for a baby?"**

Whoever got the idea that a young mother is better than an older mother has not seen the millions of mothers in their 40s and even 50s who mother with great patience, love, insight, wisdom and kindness.

This person obviously doesn't understand that with age comes maturity and wisdom.

Someone who makes a comment like this may be focusing on the energy level of children, forgetting that even most 25 year old mothers are not out playing baseball with their kids everyday.

Whoever throws out a comment about age is ignorant of the fact that a woman of any age who is ready and able to love a child, and who is brave and strong enough to endure infertility, is more prepared, capable and ready to mother than almost anyone. A good mother is a good mother, whether she is 21, 31, 41, 51 or beyond.

Dancing Your Way to Fertility is available on Amazon.com.

www.ingramcontent.com/pod-product-compliance
Lightning Source LLC
Chambersburg PA
CBHW081411280526
45788CB00009B/3052